# *A Life With Diabetes*

## A Book On Diabetes And Diabetes Management

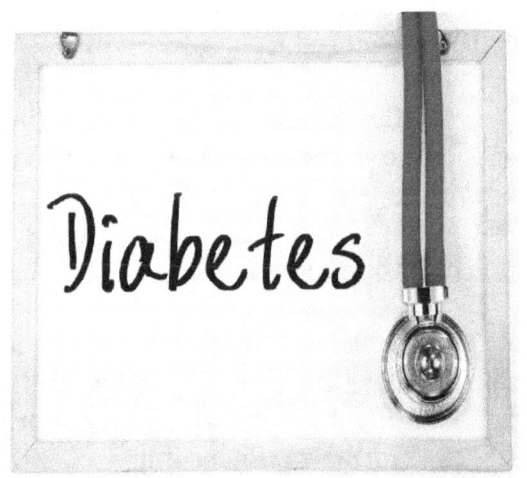

By
**Paolo Jose de Luna**

Paolo Jose De Luna

## A Life With Diabetes

The information provided herein is stated to be truthful and consistent, in that any liability, in terms of inattention or otherwise, by any usage or abuse of any policies, processes, or directions contained within is the solitary and utter responsibility of the recipient reader. Under no circumstances will any legal responsibility or blame be held against the publisher for any reparation, damages, or monetary loss due to the information herein, either directly or indirectly.

Respective authors own all copyrights not held by the publisher.

The information herein is offered for informational purposes solely, and is universal as so. The presentation of the information is without contract or any type of guarantee assurance.

The trademarks that are used are without any consent, and the publication of the trademark is without permission or backing by the trademark owner. All trademarks and brands within this book are for clarifying purposes only and are the owned by the owners themselves, not affiliated with this document.

A Life With Diabetes

# Table of Contents

# Introduction - Living With Diabetes

Diabetes mellitus is defined as a group of metabolic diseases that leads to a rise in the blood sugar levels or glucose, resulting in a condition called hyperglycemia. This may be due to a problem in the secretion of insulin, the action of insulin, or maybe even both. Glucose is normally found in the blood as a major source of nutrition for various organs, like the brain. Major sources of glucose often come from food sources that are digested through the gastrointestinal tract and formed by the liver.

Diabetes is one of the most prevalent and debilitating health problems of today. With the unstable state of the pancreas and the rising blood sugar levels of the body, several signs and symptoms take place in the body, leading to excessive thirst, hunger, and urination – the cardinal signs of diabetes. Diabetes mellitus is considered to be one of the most serious medical conditions because there's no permanent cure for it, only a lifelong management for the person to live a normal life. What's even scarier about diabetes is that it comes without warning and it comes at almost anyone. You've got that right –*anyone*. May it be man or woman, rich or poor, and even young or old, diabetes mellitus can come and develop as a potential health problem.

There are various complications that diabetes often leads to. This would include stroke, high blood pressure, liver problems, cardiovascular problems, and even amputation of one or both of your legs. You can see how diabetes can lead to life-threatening conditions despite its small beginnings. Even now, the incidence of diabetes is on the rise as most patients coming in hospitals nowadays often have diabetes mellitus on top of their main medical problem. This changes their medical treatment as certain measures are instituted to protect them from harm and to ensure that their treatment doesn't compromise their health because of the very drugs that they are given.

But alas, all is not lost. While diabetes may be a lifelong condition, there are a lot of things that you can do to manage diabetes. And for those of you who don't have this condition, there are also a lot of ways that you can do to prevent diabetes from developing in the first place. As they said before, "*Prevention is better than cure*", and when it comes to diabetes, not getting it in the first place is the best way to treat it.

This book is meant to help you, your family members, or any of your loved ones in their fight against diabetes. It doesn't mean that if you don't have diabetes, you don't have any role in their care. As a family member or a friend, you still have power to help them in their time of need, giving them information and knowledge that you can pass on to them in order to battle diabetes. In this eBook, you'll be learning all about diabetes, diabetes management, and ways on how you can prevent diabetes from developing in the first place.

# Chapter 1 - What is Diabetes?

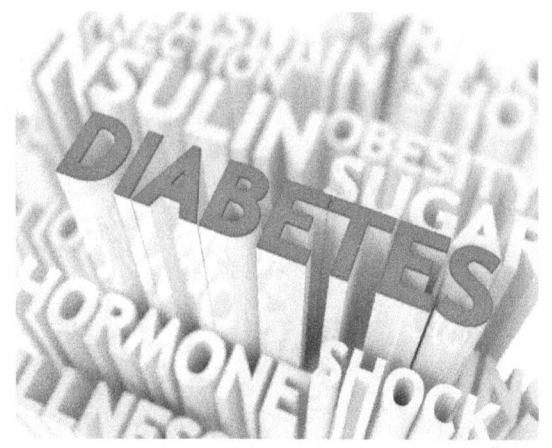

Just like winning any kind of war, the first step is to know the enemy – in this case, diabetes. Knowing diabetes in its basic sense is important to devise ways on how to handle it in the first place. It's a lifelong condition that doesn't have an immediate cure for it, but there are many ways on how to control it and how to prevent it from happening in the first place.

## A Life With Diabetes

Diabetes occurs because of a problem in the insulin secretion, in the action of the insulin, or maybe even both. Regardless of which problem may be present, this results in episodes of hyperglycemia or elevated blood glucose levels. While it's normal to have glucose in the blood since it serves as the nutrition for various organs in the body, too much glucose isn't healthy and can end up damaging the organs instead.

Insulin is produced by the pancreas and is the hormone that is responsible for controlling the glucose levels in the blood. This hormone regulates the secretion and the storage of glucose, making sure that blood sugar levels don't end up getting too high or too low. But in a diabetic person, the cells no longer respond to the effects of insulin or the pancreas doesn't produce enough insulin to control the blood glucose levels, or sometimes even both. This results in metabolic complications like diabetic ketoacidosis (DKA) or hyperglycemic hyperosmolar non-ketotic syndrome (HHNS). If left unmanaged, diabetes mellitus can result in macrovascular complications which affects the larger blood vessels like in the cases of coronary artery disease and cerebrovascular disease, microvascular complications which affects the tiny blood vessels like in the cases of kidney diseases and eye problems, and neuropathic complications which involves the nerves and can lead to nerve problems like numbness of an extremity.

## A Life With Diabetes

Diabetes affects as much as 17 million people and is still on the rise today, with about 6-7 million being undiagnosed of the condition. Diabetes mellitus is prevalent among the elderly, but can also affect the young. There are several factors that affect the development of diabetes mellitus, but most of them primarily rely on one's lifestyle habits which would include diet, exercise, smoking, sedentary lifestyle, and unhealthy habits.

The vast reach of complications that diabetes can potentially cause is what makes this lifelong condition fearsome. While it may start as mild, diabetes encompasses almost every system in the body, making a diabetic person prone to develop various health problems like myocardial infarction, coronary artery disease, stroke, cholelithiasis, pancreatitis, and a whole lot more. Today, diabetes mellitus is one of the leading causes of amputation, blindness, and renal failure.

## Risk Factors of Diabetes

There are several factors that come into play when it comes to the development of diabetes mellitus. While diabetes is said to be hereditary or passed on in the family, many of the risk factors of this lifelong condition belong to the modifiable lifestyle habits that tend to make a negative impact on one's health. The risk factors that may contribute to the development of diabetes include the following:

**A family history of diabetes**

**Obesity**

**Age (45 years old and above)**

**History of gestational diabetes**

**Previous results of impaired glucose tolerance**

**Hypertension**

**Cigarette smoking**

**Pancreatitis**

**Elevated cholesterol levels**

**Sugar-filled diet**

**Sedentary lifestyle**

Notice how the risk factors of diabetes mellitus are mostly dependent on lifestyle habits. With unhealthy lifestyle habits, you make yourself prone to develop diabetes mellitus. Today, even the younger generation is affected by diabetes, some being diagnosed as early as 25 years old. Eliminating these risk factors or taking control of them is the definite way to prevent the development of diabetes in the first place. By avoiding these risk factors, you promote your health and you have no fear in getting diabetes except for another correlated medical condition.

## The Signs and Symptoms of Diabetes

Diabetes is an endocrine and metabolic disorder that encompasses almost every system in the body. It can reach the cardiovascular system, the nervous system, the musculoskeletal system, and even the renal system. This makes diabetes mellitus an incredibly frightening disease that has no cure and is lifelong, often detected late because of its onset. Because of this, you should know the common signs and symptoms that diabetic people exhibit to administer the proper care in the earliest time, especially when it's already turned into an emergency situation. It's usually when hyperglycemia kicks in that these signs and symptoms start to show up. Here are some of the signs and symptoms of diabetes that you need to watch out for:

**Polyuria or increased urination**

**Polydipsia or increased thirst**

**Polyphagia or increased hunger**

**Elevated blood sugar levels**

**Weakness**

**Visual changes**

**Tingling or numbness in the hands or feet**

**Dry skin**

**Wounds or skin lesions that are not healing or healing too slowly**

**Recurrent infections**

**Weight loss**

**Nausea**

**Vomiting**

**Abdominal pain**

The three main symptoms of diabetes include the 3 Ps – polyuria, polydipsia, and polyphagia. These three symptoms result from the fluid loss that occurs in diabetes through osmosis and the catabolic state that the cells undergo during a diabetic state. The other signs and symptoms result from the consequences of raised blood sugar level to the blood vessels, causing macrovascular, microvascular, and neuropathic changes. Because glucose has a role in every vital organ, you'll also notice a myriad of signs and symptoms associated with the damaged organ like renal failure, numbness of the extremities, or even increase the likelihood of a stroke.

## The Complications of Diabetes

When diabetes is left to freely run its course, it can lead to a number of complications that can range from short term problems up to lifelong and chronic conditions that need to be managed on top of diabetes. Since glucose has a role in supplying nutrients to every organ system, you'll notice how the complications cover almost every system. This is how important controlling blood sugar is and without adequate control over the production and the action of insulin, it can lead to serious complications. Here are just some that you need to take note of:

**Hypoglycemia or decreased blood sugar levels**

**Diabetic Ketoacidosis (DKA)**

**Hyperglycemic Hyperosmolar Non-ketotic Syndrome (HHNS)**

**Atherosclerosis**

**Coronary artery disease**

**Myocardial infarction or heart attack**

**Cerebrovascular disease**

**Peripheral vascular disease**

**Diabetic foot disease**

**Diabetic retinopathy**

**Cataracts**

**Lens Damage**

**Extraocular muscle palsy**

**Glaucoma**

**Nephropathy**

**End Stage Renal Disease (ESRD)**

**Renal failure**

**Diabetic neuropathy**

**Neuropathic ulcers**

**Recurring infections**

The complications of diabetes mellitus are certainly scary. Most of them are even lifelong conditions, requiring you to manage them as long as you live, increasing your medical expenses on treatment, hospitalization, and medications. However, all of this can be prevented by observing the proper measures of controlling diabetes and preventing diabetes from developing in the first place. Getting to know these complications is crucial to be able to know what to do when they start to develop and to detect them early on so that treatment can be started without any delay.

It's true – diabetes sounds scary. And there's no blaming you if you're starting to feel afraid of it. But fear not, as there are various ways on how to prevent diabetes and even how to control it once you are diagnosed with it. Lifestyle is what plays a crucial factor in diabetes, whether in preventing it or in controlling it. It's what you do with your life and what habits you adapt that are important. But know what diabetes is firsthand and how to identify it are the keys to establish the proper interventions and measures on how to fight it or to help anyone who has diabetes, whether it's a friend, a family member, or a loved one.

The management of diabetes relies on five main factors – diet, exercise, blood glucose monitoring, pharmacologic therapy, and education. After getting yourself educated about diabetes mellitus, it's time to tackle the rest of the factors involved in managing diabetes.

# Chapter 2 - The Diabetic Diet

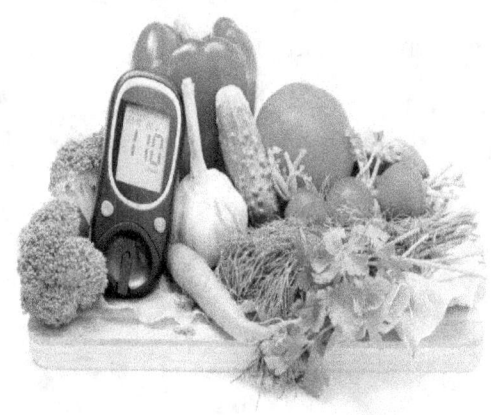

After getting to know more about diabetes, it's time to learn on how to manage it. The first step that we're going to talk about is diet and it's one of the biggest factors that a diabetic needs to be knowledgeable of since it's one of the easiest to modify. If diet is not taken into consideration, controlling blood sugar levels can be difficult to do.

# A Life With Diabetes

A healthy diet is a key to healthy living, whether or not you have diabetes. But if you are a diabetic, then a healthy diet will be your lifeline that will save you from the various complications that diabetes can bring. And when it comes to a healthy diet, it's not just what kinds of food that you eat that matter, you also have to think about how much food you eat and the combinations of food that you eat.

Taking into account what you eat is a crucial factor to control and to prevent diabetes from ever happening in the first place. Ensuring that your blood glucose levels are within normal limits may sound like a challenge, but it's more of placing discipline to one's self rather than totally restricting food from your diet. Here are some of the important factors that you need to take note of when it comes to managing your diet and controlling your blood sugar levels:

**Learn to Count Carbs** – When it comes to diabetes management, counting calories and carbohydrates is important. It's carbohydrates that have a bigger impact on your blood sugar levels because they're sugar that are readily used by the body. For those on insulin therapy, it's important that you know about the amount of carbohydrates that you take in for every meal to adjust the dosage of your insulin and ensure that you don't get too little or too much insulin.

**Portions and Sizes** – Planning the portions of your meals in advance is helpful when it comes to managing your diabetic diet. You can use scales or measuring cups to ensure that you get adequate nutrition while also getting in control of your carb intake. This way, you can also eat what you want to eat without depriving yourself of delicious food – just at the proper portions and sizes.

A Balanced Meal – Making every meal balanced is a key in managing your blood sugar levels when it comes to your diet. As much as you can, include a good combination of fruits, vegetables, proteins, starches, and fats to your diet. Getting a hand in measuring portions and sizes helps here since you have to plan your meals in advance. And if you're already got the basics down, you'll be surprised at how much food that you can eat and the kinds of food that you can eat in a balanced diet. If you want more advice on your diet, you can consult your physician or dietician to learn more on what kinds of food that you can include in your balanced meal.

**Timing Meals with Meds** – If you eat too little and you still have to take your anti-diabetic medications, it can result in a dangerously low blood sugar level or hypoglycemia. However, too much food may lead you to have an increased blood sugar level or hyperglycemia. Talk with your doctor on how to time your meals and medications, especially insulin, so that you won't suffer the consequences when it comes to the dose and schedule of your meals and medications.

A Life With Diabetes

**No Sugary or Sweetened Drinks** – A fan of sodas or carbonated drinks? Well, if you have diabetes, you have to accept that they're bad for you and you should avoid them as much as possible. These drinks are excessively sweetened with high fructose corn syrup or sucrose, giving you a high amount of calories but too little when it comes to nutrition. They cause blood sugar levels to rise quickly and if you're diabetic, it's best to avoid these beverages. In fact, if you want to avoid getting diabetes, you have to learn on how to avoid these drinks. The only exception is here is that when you're experiencing an excessively low blood sugar level or hypoglycemia, you can take any of these drinks, like soda or juice, to serve as an emergency treatment to raise the blood sugar levels.

Diet is always an essential factor when it comes to managing diabetes. It plays a huge role when it comes to controlling blood sugar since food is our primary source of nutrition and that's where we get our sugars from. Of course, it's already a given that we need that sugar to function properly since the vital organs, like the brain, use glucose as their source of nutrition. However, too much glucose can be deadly, most especially for diabetics. If you want to manage your blood sugar levels properly, then the kind, the amount, and the combination of food that you eat certainly matters.

A healthy and balanced diet doesn't just help in controlling diabetes. It will also help prevent the development of other health problems like heart disease, stroke, gastrointestinal problems, and more. You also get the chance to lose weight since you'll be eating what you need and when you need it, focusing mostly on fruits and vegetables, as well as starch sources on top of proteins and fats.

Getting engaged in a faithful diet regimen is often the biggest challenge for many people, whether or not they have diabetes. But when it comes to diet, investing time, money, patience, hard work, and discipline is important so you can take this crucial first step towards losing weight, controlling diabetes, or maybe just towards a healthy lifestyle.

# Chapter 3 - Getting More Exercise

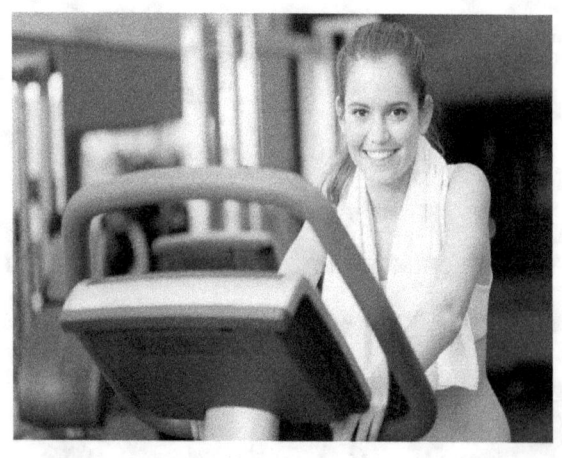

When it comes to a healthy lifestyle, diet and exercise go well in tandem together. That crucial combination never disappears and it never will when it comes to promoting good health. In fact, most health conditions recommend that you get adequate exercise to prevent them from developing. This is why exercise is so important when it comes to our health. Just next to diet, exercise also places equal importance when it comes to managing diabetes.

Physical activity allows your muscle to use up glucose to build up energy. Regular exercise helps your body use up sugar, therefore promoting the use of insulin in a much more efficient manner. As these mechanisms work together, your blood sugar level is kept at a constant level, making it easier to control your blood sugar even when you're a diabetic.

However, it's not just about going to the gym or going out on a run – regular physical activity like gardening, doing housework, walking, and doing chores can help improve and control your blood glucose levels. Here are the things that you can do to when it comes to your exercise:

**Devising an Exercise Plan** – If you want to build an exercise regimen from scratch, you can ask your doctor about it since you need to know what kind of physical activities are suited for you. Most adults should exercise at least 30 minutes every day, about 5 days a week. If it's been a long time since you've last exercised, you might want to have your general health checked out by your doctor before even doing any kind of exercise. After assessing your condition, you and your doctor can talk about building your exercise plan and maintaining a good balance of cardio and strength exercises.

# A Life With Diabetes

**Sticking to a Schedule** – After building your exercise regimen, it's time to set your schedule for your exercise so that you can follow through. You can ask your physician about the best time of the day for your exercise so that your meals and your medications work in a synergistic manner with your exercise. Setting a schedule ensures that your glucose levels are at a balanced state, preventing episodes of excessive blood sugar levels or depleted blood sugar levels.

**Knowing the Numbers** – Before even beginning your exercise regimen, you should first ask your doctor regarding the safety margins for you to start working out. Ask about the safest blood sugar values that you are allowed to exercise to prevent events of decreased blood sugar levels.

**Checking Your Blood Sugar** – It's important that you check your blood sugar levels before physical activity, during exercise, and then after working out. If you're on insulin therapy or taking oral anti-diabetic agents, knowing your blood sugar levels is important. Exercising lowers the blood sugar levels by making use of the glucose in the body to be used as energy and having an already low blood sugar level can further decreased it. If you notice that your blood sugar level is below normal or just borderline lower values of the normal blood sugar level, then having a small snack before exercising is important. Subsequently, if you notice signs and symptoms of hypoglycemia (shakiness, weakness, hunger, thirst, fatigue, lightheadedness, irritability, anxiety, confusion, etc.) during or after exercise, you might need to take something that has a high calorie content like a soda or juice to give you a boost of energy that you need.

**Drink Plenty of Water** – Prevent getting dehydrated by drinking plenty of water while you exercise. That's because dehydration can also affect blood sugar levels, worsening the signs and symptoms of hypoglycemia which can lead to serious complications if left untreated.

**Being Prepared** – If you're going out to exercise, always have a small snack like a cookie or a sports drink as a good source of energy in any case that your blood sugar levels start to drop too low. Also wear your medical identification band or bracelet to indicate that you're diabetic in any case that you collapse or lose consciousness, so that people or emergency responders know what to do with you to help you regain consciousness.

## Adjunct Planning with Medications

– If you're on insulin therapy, you may need to adjust your dose or your timing so that you won't experience hypoglycemic reactions while you exercise. Be sure to ask your doctor about this so that he can adjust your medications for you, especially before you go out and workout.

## A Life With Diabetes

Developing an exercise regimen may sound hard, but it's quite an enjoyable experience that will teach you on how to manage your own time and it will help you work hard towards your goal. An individualized exercise regimen is the best for diabetics since the regular cardio and strength exercises may already be too much or even too little for some people. This is also why it's important to get the second opinion of someone you trust just like your physician or maybe even a close family member.

Physical activity changes everything when it comes to diabetes management. Just like diet, you need to invest time and patience with it, requiring you to plan out your exercise regimens and what kind of physical activities that you can do.

Diabetes management is a reachable goal with effort and patience, leading you to engage in healthy lifestyle habits and getting enough exercise is just one of them.

# Chapter 4 - Monitoring and Medications

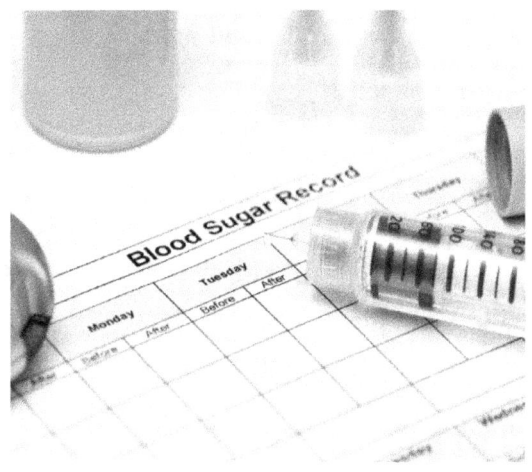

Diet and exercise certainly play big roles when it comes to managing diabetes. However, it's not just about engaging in healthy lifestyle habits that you can manage diabetes. There are times when diet and exercise might not just be enough in controlling your blood sugar levels.

When it comes to the more active aspect of controlling blood sugar levels, anti-diabetic medications play a vital role and monitoring your blood glucose on a routine basis is a must to know your blood sugar and prevent any cases of hyperglycemia or hypoglycemia.

Insulin is just one of the many anti-diabetic medications for those with diabetes mellitus. This hormone controls the blood sugar levels by allowing the cells to use the glucose in the blood and insulin often comes in an injectable form. Other anti-diabetic medications in the form of tablets are also available which help reduce the blood sugar levels, albeit at a slower rate since they need to be digested by the stomach and absorbed by the intestines.

Do note that the effectiveness of these anti-diabetic medications depend on the timing that they are administered and the dose of the medication. Here are some of the things that you need to remember when it comes to your anti-diabetic medications and monitoring your blood glucose levels:

**StoringInsulin** – Insulin should be stored properly so that it doesn't get wasted. Often coming in vials or insulin pen injections, insulin should be stored in a cool place like in the refrigerator, but should not be frozen. This prevents the decay of the medication and can be used for a long time. Be sure that you check the expiration date of the insulin before you can administer it.

**Monitoring Your Blood Sugar Levels –** Buying a blood glucose machine to measure your blood sugar levels on a routine basis is helpful so that you'll know when to take your emergency anti-diabetic medications and to manage your diet, exercise, and medications properly. Today, blood glucose machines aren't that expensive and they often come with lancets for getting blood samples and blood sugar strips that can measure your blood sugar levels.

**Rotating Injection Sites –** If you're taking injectable insulin on a routine basis, you need to rotate your injection sites to prevent hardening of the skin. Lipodystrophy is the abnormal hardening of the skin, particularly in the injection sites that are repeatedly pierced by needles. To prevent this, you need to transfer injection sites routinely, for example, injecting on the left upper arms first, then the right upper arms, then the abdomen, then the left thigh, and then the right thigh.

**Always on Time** – When it comes to anti-diabetic medications, timing is always important. You shouldn't miss out on the schedule of your medications to prevent sudden episodes of hyperglycemia or hypoglycemia that often occur for those who don't follow their anti-diabetic medication regimen.

**Needles and Injections** – Insulin often comes as in an injectable form. Because of how insulin is administered, using a new insulin syringe is important to prevent infections on the injection site. For the pre-filled insulin pens, you can change the needle tips easily and they're replaced with a new one that's sterile and ready to be used.

**Be Wary of New Medications** – If you're thinking about taking a new medication, whether it's for your diabetes or for other health problems, be sure to consult your physician because these medications may have certain effects to your blood sugar levels which can potentially trigger episodes of hypoglycemia or hyperglycemia.

**Consulting Your Physician** – If you notice that your blood glucose levels often get too low or too high, consult your physician immediately. This may be because that your medications may not have the adequate dose or have the right timing, triggering your blood sugar levels to become unstable.

The medications in diabetes play a vital role in controlling the blood sugar levels on an active basis. When diet and exercise don't seem to be enough to control the blood sugar, that's when anti-diabetic medications kick in. Monitoring your blood sugar is also important so that you can take note of episodes of hyperglycemia and hypoglycemia, and take your anti-diabetic medications on time and with the right dosage. It's important that you should be knowledgeable when it comes to anti-diabetic medications since they are often lifelong, but you shouldn't just rely on your medications in controlling your blood sugars. Despite the powerful effect of anti-diabetic medications, eating a healthy diet and getting adequate exercise are important to maintain a constant level of blood sugar that's within normal limits and prevent the various complications of diabetes to develop.

# CONCLUSION

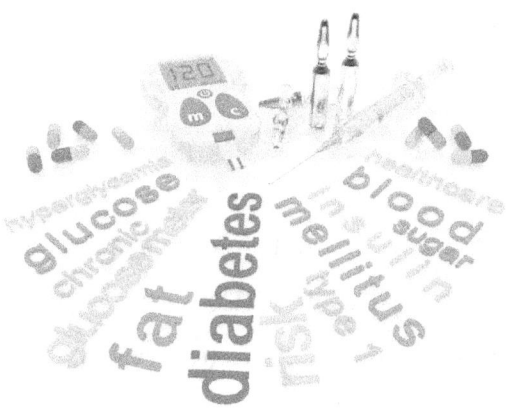

Diabetes affects millions of people worldwide. In fact, there are a lot of people with diabetes who go undiagnosed, leaving it already too late for them once the signs and symptoms or even the complications show up. Diabetes mellitus encompasses almost all organ systems in the body, bringing a myriad of signs and symptoms that can debilitate anyone, regardless of race, age, or origin.

But despite the life-threatening complications and lifelong status of diabetes mellitus, all is not yet lost as there are ways on managing this metabolic disorder.

Diet is the first one that plays a role in managing diabetes. With a healthy diet, diabetes is not just controlled, it can also be prevented from happening in the first place, stopping it in its tracks before it could even begin. A healthy diet is comprised mostly of vegetables and fruits, along with good sources of starch, proteins, and fats. And it's not just diabetes that a healthy diet can prevent – it can also prevent the development of other health problems like heart attacks, coronary artery disease, stroke, renal disease, and a lot more.

## A Life With Diabetes

Getting enough exercise also helps in managing diabetes because physical activity reduces the buildup of glucose in the blood. With increased physical demand, the body makes use of glucose to produce energy, effectively preventing the episodes of hyperglycemia. This also helps the action of the insulin to kick in since the toll for the hormone to control the blood sugar is reduced because the body is making use of some of the glucose for energy. Exercise is also a gateway intervention to achieve weight loss, further helping out in the management of diabetes.

Anti-diabetic medications work together with diet and exercise, providing a more active way to control blood sugar. These medications serve as the lifeline when eating a healthy and balanced diet, and getting enough exercise aren't enough to control the blood sugar levels. Consulting your physician is important when it comes to determining the dosage, the timing, and building the entire schedule of your anti-diabetic medications and utmost loyalty to the medication regimen is important to prevent cases of rebound hyperglycemia and resistance to the administered insulin. Most people often have a denial when it comes to this stage, refusing that taking anti-diabetic medications is a lifelong ordeal. However, you have to learn and accept that this is just the way that it's going to be since diabetes mellitus is a chronic condition that needs to be managed constantly.

## A Life With Diabetes

Sure, a life with diabetes may sound difficult and depressing. Diabetes mellitus is a lifelong condition without any sort of cure. However, that doesn't mean that you should just pack up and give up all together. Managing diabetes is possible through controlling the blood sugar levels. Diabetes management relies on several factors like eating a healthy diet, getting enough exercise, educating one's self about diabetes, learning about your anti-diabetic medications, and monitoring your blood glucose on a daily basis.

It can certainly be a challenge. You'll need to invest time, money, and a whole lot of effort when it comes to managing diabetes. It's not going to be an easy task, but it's a rewarding one for sure.

If you have a family member, a friend, or a loved one who has diabetes, it's going to be your job to teach them about this disease. Or if you do have diabetes, it's going to be okay and you'll manage just fine after learning everything about managing diabetes in this eBook.